Human Anatomy for Kids

By: Keerthana Madireddi

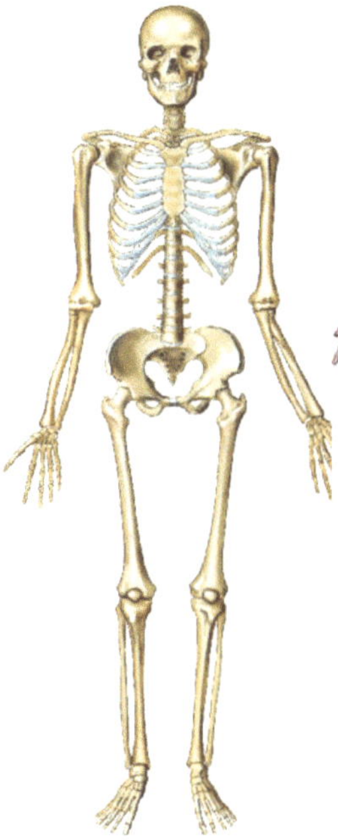

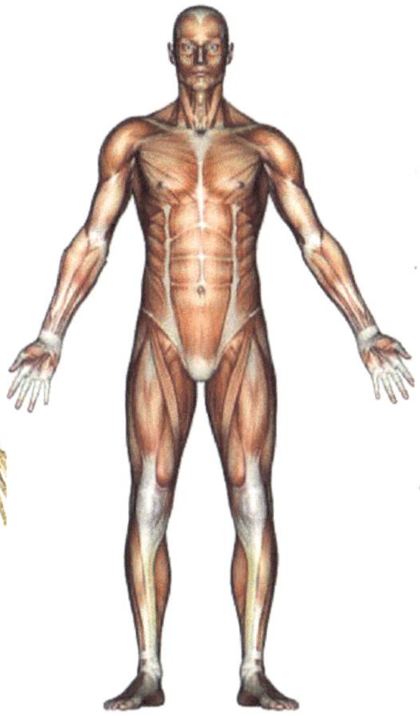

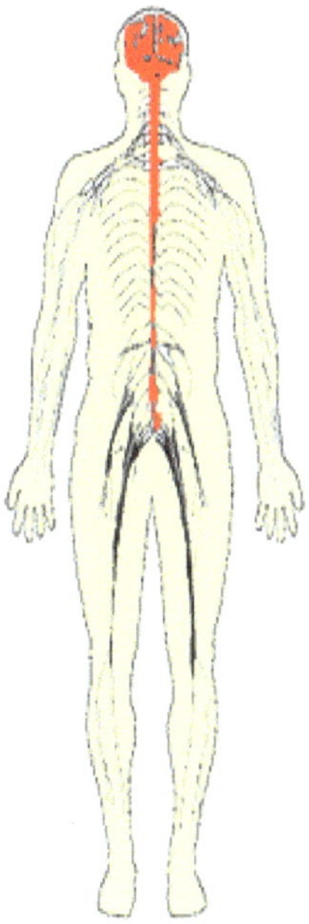

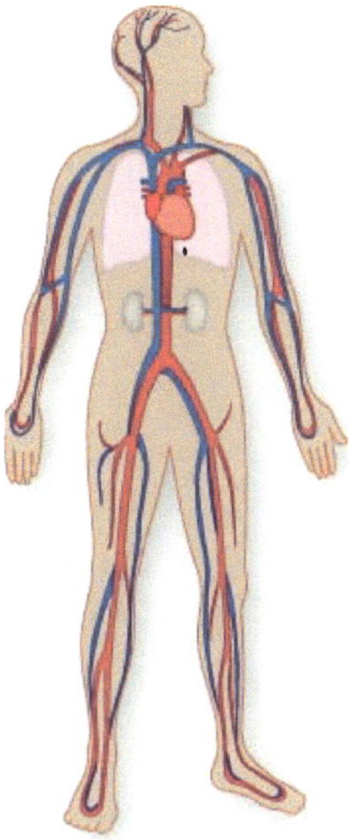

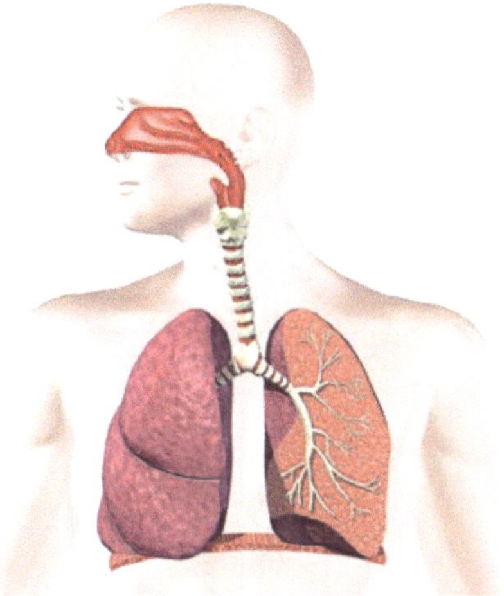

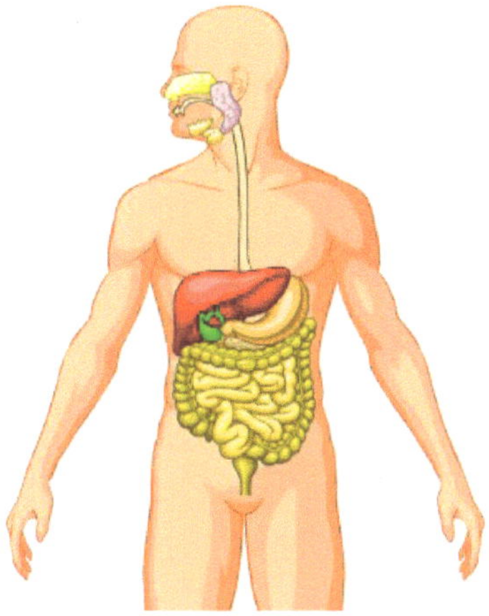

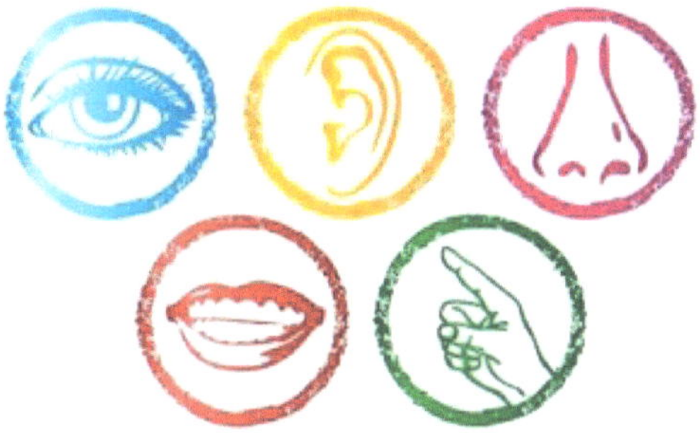

Hi! This is a resource that was prepared for middle level students to learn about human anatomy, with added fun facts and functions.
The booklet is divided into sections that represent some of the major body systems.

Table of Contents

The Basics

Cells

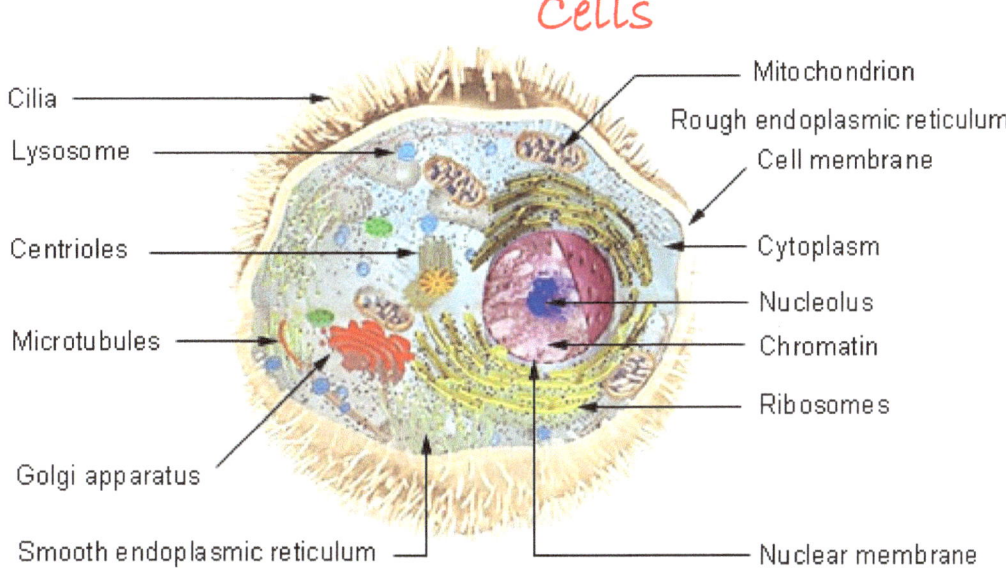

Cilia — Mitochondrion

Lysosome — Rough endoplasmic reticulum

— Cell membrane

Centrioles — Cytoplasm

— Nucleolus

Microtubules — Chromatin

— Ribosomes

Golgi apparatus

Smooth endoplasmic reticulum — Nuclear membrane

http://people.eku.edu/ritchisong/301notes1.htm

Parts of a cell and their function

➢ Cilia: moves the cell around; acts like wheels; tiny hair
➢ Lysosomes: clean the cell; acts like janitor
➢ Mitochondrion: supply cell with energy; acts like the power plant
➢ Rough and Smooth Endoplasmic Reticulum: assemble proteins; acts like the assembly
➢ Cell Membrane: separates the cell from others; gives cell its shape; acts like boundaries
➢ Centrioles: divides cells; acts like a factory
➢ Microtubules: move proteins to different parts of the cell; acts like a delivery truck
➢ Cytoplasm: thick fluid outside the nucleus and inside the cell membrane; acts like a skeleton of the cell
➢ Nucleus: the oval part with the nucleolus, chromatin, and nuclear membrane; controls the cells; acts like the government; located in the center
➢ Chromatin and Nucleolus: contains genetic information(DNA and RNA); acts like a document
➢ Nuclear membrane: boundary for the nucleus; acts like boundaries
➢ Golgi Apparatus: help package protein; acts like packaging factory
➢ Ribosome: help make protein; acts like grocery store

Fun Facts about a cell

➢ Many cells make up a tissue; many tissues make up an organ; many organs make up a system; many systems make up your body
➢ One human cell contains 46 chromosomes
➢ You have approximately 100 trillion cells in your body
➢ A typical cell is 10 micrometers in size and 1 nanogram in mass
➢ Cells contain structures called organelles which carry out specific functions
➢ Cells have varying life spans

DNA

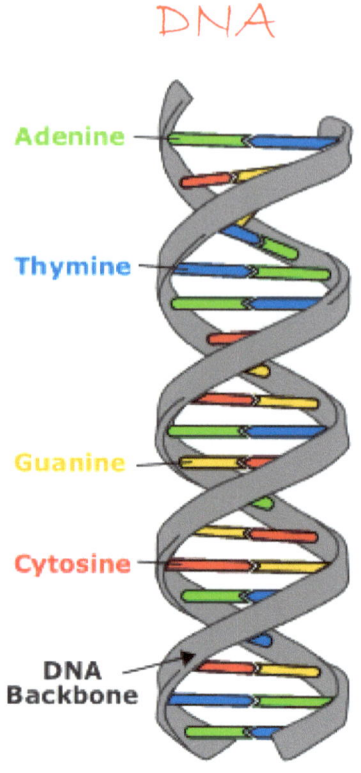

http://evolution.berkeley.edu/evolibrary/article/mutations_02

Parts of a DNA and their cell and function

➢ Adenine: the energy or fuel of the DNA; pairs wiht thymine; contains code for DNA
➢ Thymine: pairs with adenine; contains a code for DNA
➢ Guanine: pairs with cytosine; contains code for DNA
➢ Cytosine: pairs with guanine; contains code for DNA
➢ DNA backbone:made out of sugar; holds the DNA together

Fun Facts about a DNA

➢ DNA stands for deoxyribonucleic acid
➢ RNA stands for Ribonucleic Acid
➢ DNA structure is called double helix
➢ RNA is a single helix
➢ If you put all the DNA molecules in your body end to end, the DNA would reach from the Earth to the Sun and back over 600 times
➢ You have 98% of your DNA in common with a chimpanzee
➢ Humans and cabbage share about 40-50% common DNA
➢ Friedrich Miescher discovered DNA in 1869, although scientists did not understand DNA was the genetic material in cells until 1943. Before that time, it was widely believe that proteins stored genetic information

Tissues

Types of tissues

➤ Epithelial: protects your body from moisture loss, bacteria, and internal injury; 2 types:
  a) Covering and lining epithelium covers or lines almost all of your internal and external body surfaces; for example, the outermost layer of your skin and other organs
  b) Glandular epithelium secretes hormones or other products such as stomach acid, sweat, saliva, and milk
➤ Connective: provides structure and support to the body; 2 types:
  c) Loose connective tissue holds structures together; for example, loose connective tissue holds the outer layer of skin to the underlying muscle tissue
  d) Fibrous connective tissue also holds body parts together; found in ligaments, cartilage, and bone
➤ Nervous: forms the nervous system
➤ Muscular: contracts; 3 types
  a) Skeletal muscle is attached to bones and causes movements of the body
  b) Cardiac muscle is found in the heart
  c) Smooth muscle lines the walls of blood vessels and certain organs

Fun Facts about tissues

➤ Cartilage is one of the few tissues that grows throughout life. Between ages 30 and 70, a nose might grow half an inch, and the ears grow about a quarter of an inch
➤ There are more than 600 individual skeletal muscles

Tissue Repair

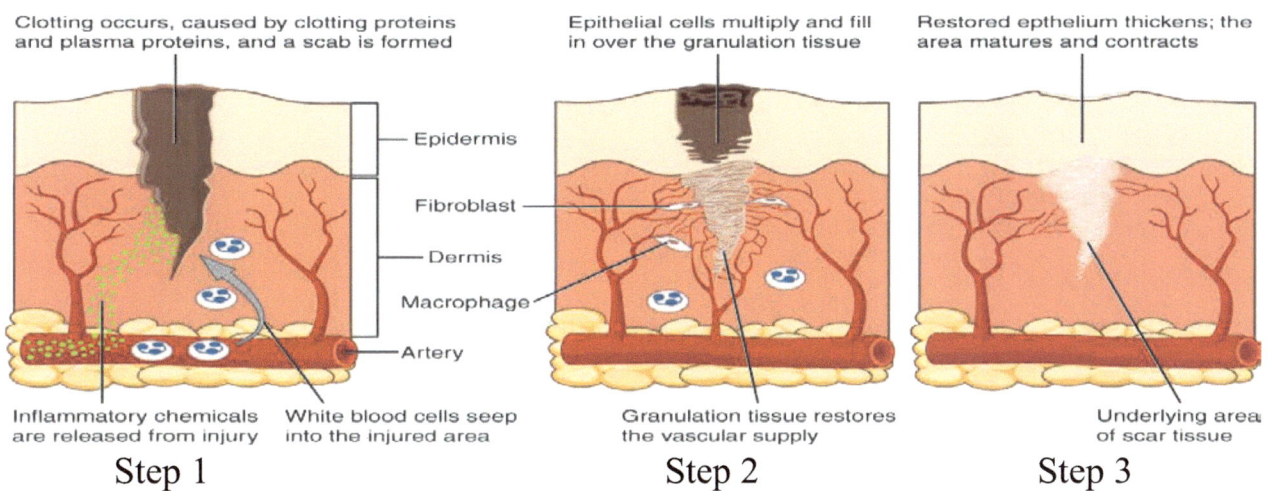

Clotting occurs, caused by clotting proteins and plasma proteins, and a scab is formed

Epithelial cells multiply and fill in over the granulation tissue

Restored epthelium thickens; the area matures and contracts

Epidermis
Fibroblast
Dermis
Macrophage
Artery

Inflammatory chemicals are released from injury
White blood cells seep into the injured area
Step 1

Granulation tissue restores the vascular supply
Step 2

Underlying area of scar tissue
Step 3

http://cnx.org/content/m46058/latest/?collection=col11496/latest

Sweat

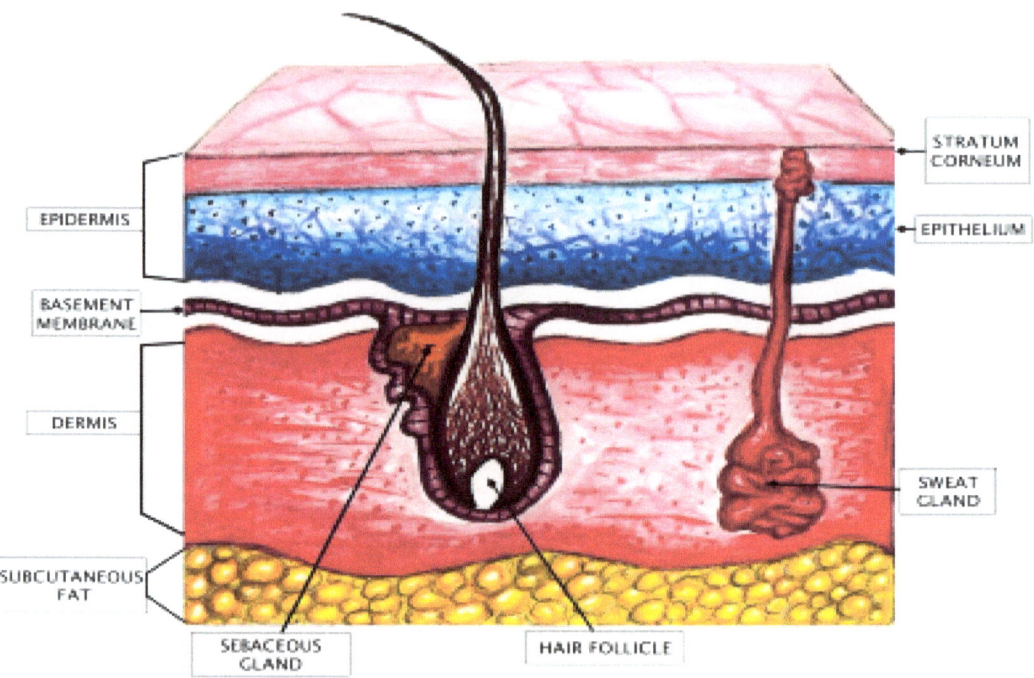

http://www.examiner.com/article/hyperhidrosis-how-to-deal-with-excessive-sweating

How you sweat

➢ Evaporation causes the sweat to release from glands

Why you sweat

➢ To get rid of heat
➢ Another way of getting rid of waste

Fun Facts about sweat

➢ The average person has 2.6 million sweat glands in their body
➢ Your feet have over 250,000 sweat glands
➢ Sometimes your body makes sweat even when in cool temperatures. This is known as insensible perspiration
➢ Only mammals have sweat glands

Skin, Hair, and Nails

Structure

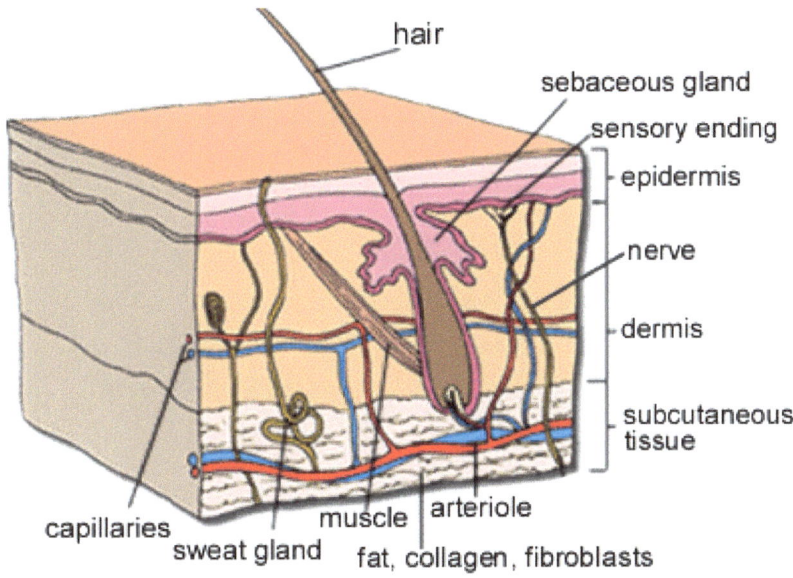

http://www.nku.edu/~dempseyd/SKIN.htm

Parts of the skin and its function

- The epidermis: the outermost layer of skin; provides a waterproof barrier; creates our skin tone
- The dermis: beneath the epidermis; contains tough connective tissue, hair follicles, and sweat glands
- The deeper subcutaneous tissue :hypodermis; made up of fat and connective tissue
- Sebaceous gland: produces sebum , a type of natural oil produced by your body, that protects your skin for being dry
- Subcutaneous fat: contains not only fatty tissues but also blood vessels, which supply the skin with oxygen, and nerves

Fun Facts about skin

- The human body's largest organ
- Is thickest on the palms of your hands and soles of your feet (around 1.5mm thick)
- When stretched out it is 2 square meters and weighs 8-10 lbs
- Is thinnet on eyelids (.02 mm thick)
- Loses about 30,000 to 40,000 dead skin cells from the surface almost every minute
- Goose bumps help retain a layer of warm air over your body
- Measures about 1 mm thick at birth and grows to about 2-3 mm thick by adulthood
- Each 5 square cm of skin may have up to 600 sweat glands

Skin color

Fun Facts about skin color

➢ Skin color is the result of melonin
➢ Skin comes in different colors throughout the world
➢ About 7% of skin cells is melonin
➢ 2 types of melonin: pheomelonin ranges from yellow to red color and eumelonin ranges from dark brown to black
➢ Everybody has the same umber of melocytes; color is resulted by activity not quantity
➢ 1 in 110,000 people have ablinism, which is no color
➢ Eye color is also resulted by melonin
➢ It takes 6 months for a baby to have permanent skin color

Hair

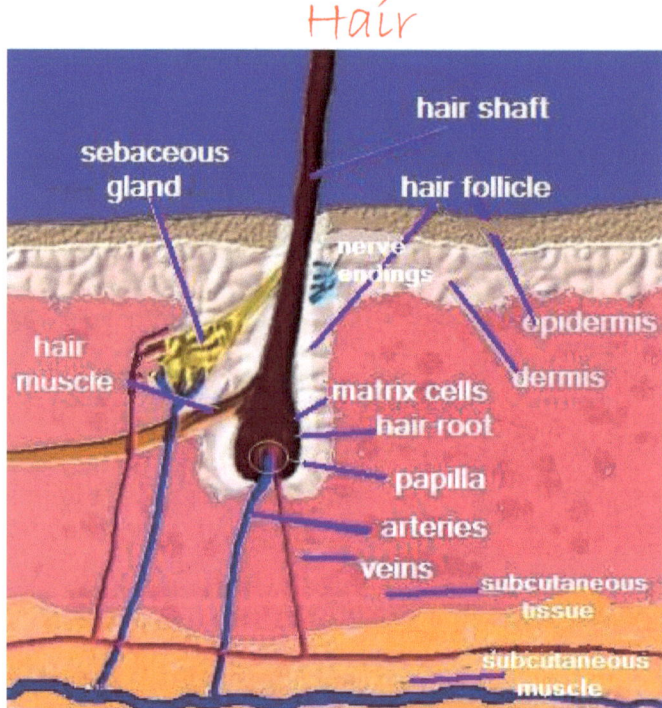

http://healthfavo.com/hair-diagram-structure.html

Fun Facts about hair

➢ Made up of keratin
➢ You lose about 20-100 hairs per day
➢ Female hair grows slower than male hair
➢ After bone marrow, hair is the fastest growing tissue
➢ Male hair is more dense than female hair
➢ Hair grows faster in warm weather
➢ Average scalp has 100,000 hairs
➢ 90% of scalp hairs are growing and 10% are resting

Nails

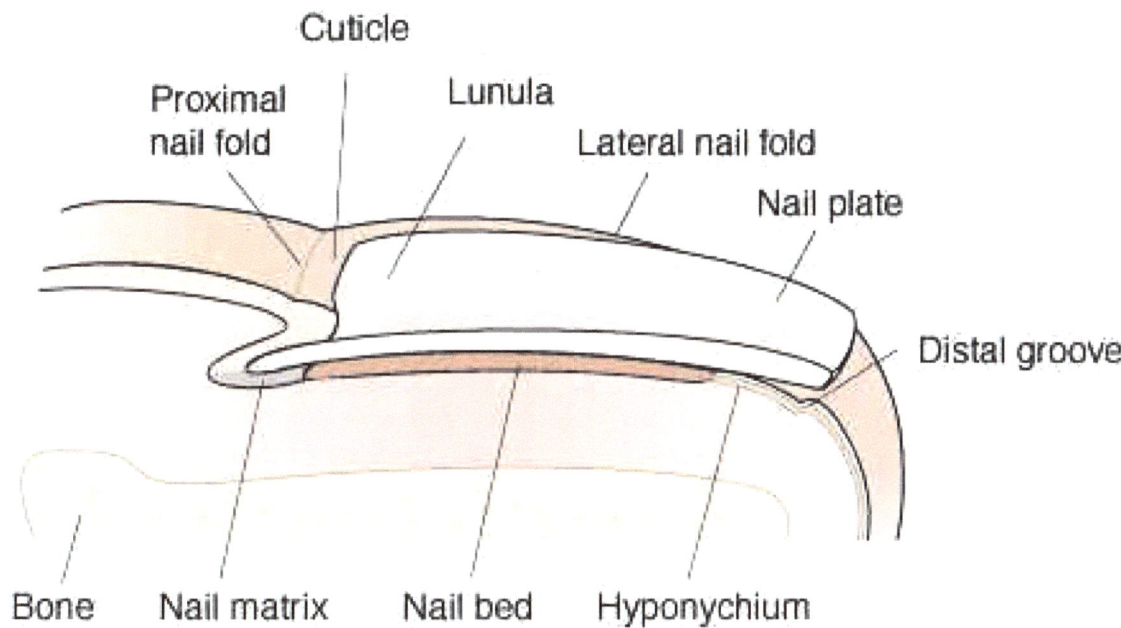

Cuticle

Proximal nail fold

Lunula

Lateral nail fold

Nail plate

Distal groove

Bone   Nail matrix   Nail bed   Hyponychium

http://www.footdoc.ca/Website%20Nail%20Conditions%20(A%20Glossary).htm

Fun Facts about nails

- ➢ Male nails grow faster than female nails
- ➢ Your finger nails(1 cm for every 100 days) grow faster than your toe nails(1 cm for about 12 to 18 months)
- ➢ Toe nails are twice as thick as finger nails
- ➢ Fastest growing nail is on the middle finger; slowest is thumb nail
- ➢ Grow faster in summers and warmer conditions; grows faster during the day than night

Skeletal System
Main Bones

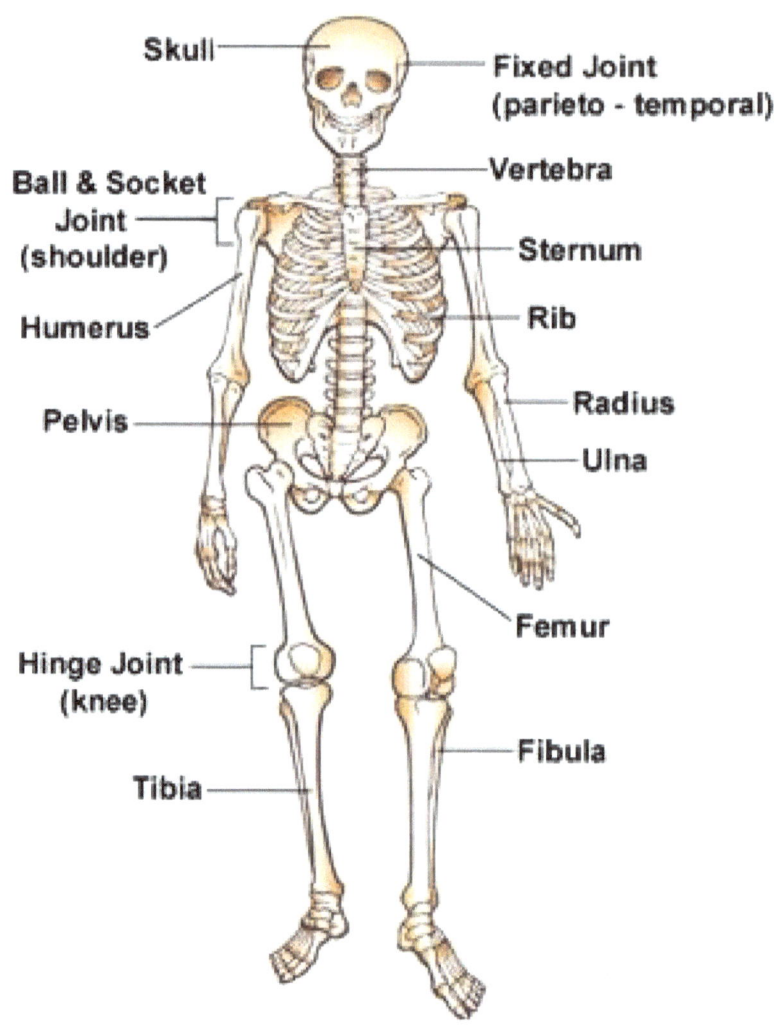

Skull — Fixed Joint (parieto - temporal)

Ball & Socket Joint (shoulder) — Vertebra

Humerus — Sternum

Pelvis — Rib

Radius

Ulna

Hinge Joint (knee) — Femur

Tibia — Fibula

http://questgarden.com/84/76/9/090714174605/

Fun Facts about bones

➢ You have more than 300 bones when you are born, but an adult has 206 bones
➢ Most of your bones are in your hands! You have 50 in your wrist
➢ Your face has 14 bones
➢ The longest bone in your body is your thigh bone or femur. It is 1/4 of your body height
➢ The smallest bones is the stirup in the ear. It 1/10 of an inch
➢ People and giraffes have the same amount of bones in the neck. The bones of a giraffe are just bigger

Joints

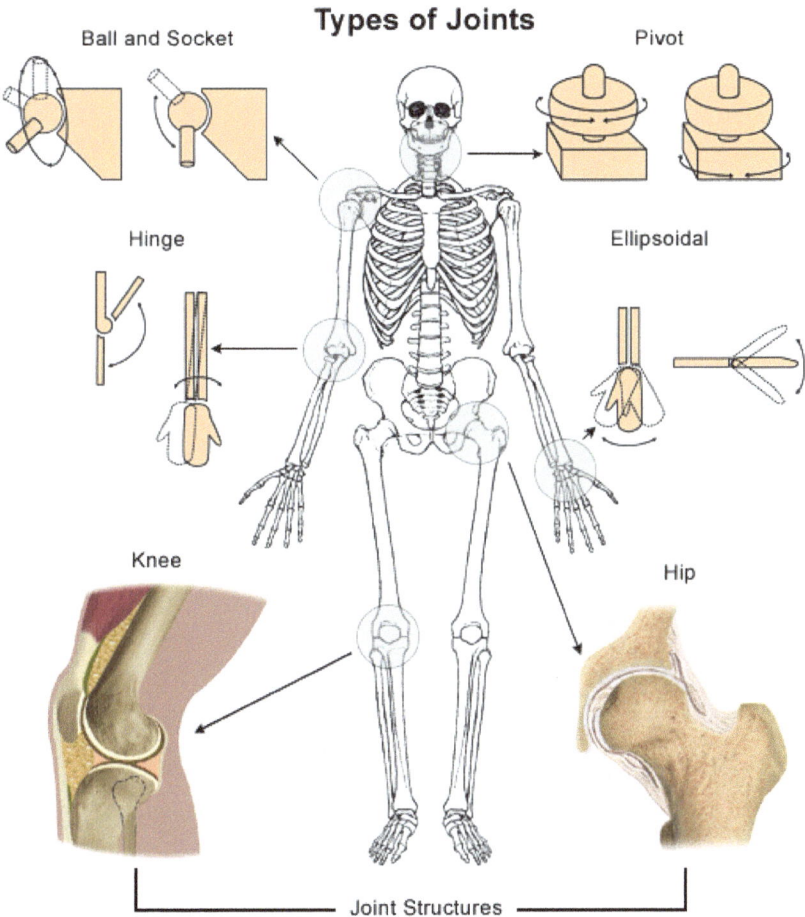

http://www.answering-christianity.com/360_joints.htm

Types of joints

➢ Ball and socket: shoulder and hip
➢ Pivot: neck
➢ Hinge: elbow and knee
➢ Ellipsoidal: wrist and ankle

Fun Facts about joints

➢ Ligaments are short bands of tough fibrous connective tissue that function to connect one bone to another, forming the joint
➢ Tendons are made of elastic tissue and also play a key role in the functioning of joints; connect muscle to bones
➢ Cartilage covers the bone surface and keeps the bones from rubbing directly against each other
➢ Ball and socket joints are the most mobile type of joint
➢ Joints in your skull don't move because they are immovable
➢ immovable joints are only found in your skull and ribs

Structure

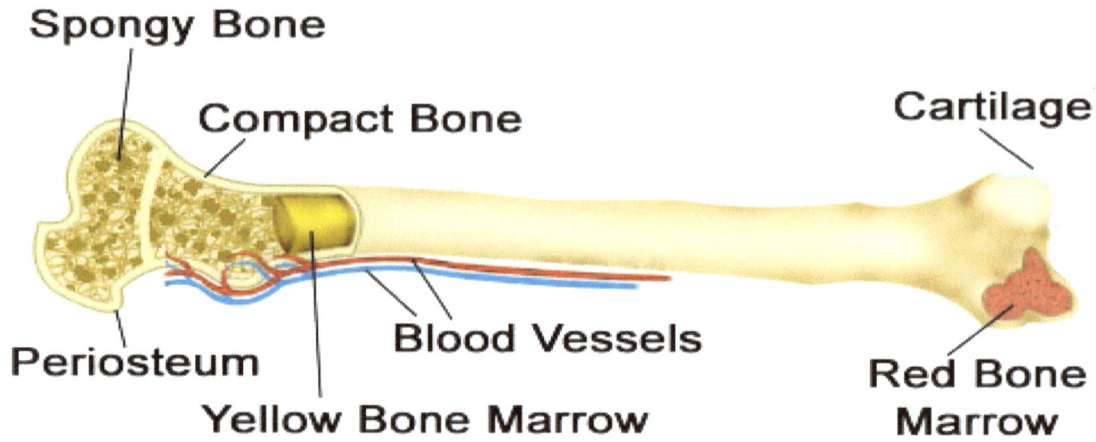

Fun Facts about bone structure

➤ Every second, your bone marrow produces two million red blood cells
➤ Made up of calcium, phosphorus, sodium, and other minerals, as well as the protein collagen

Muscular System
Main muscles

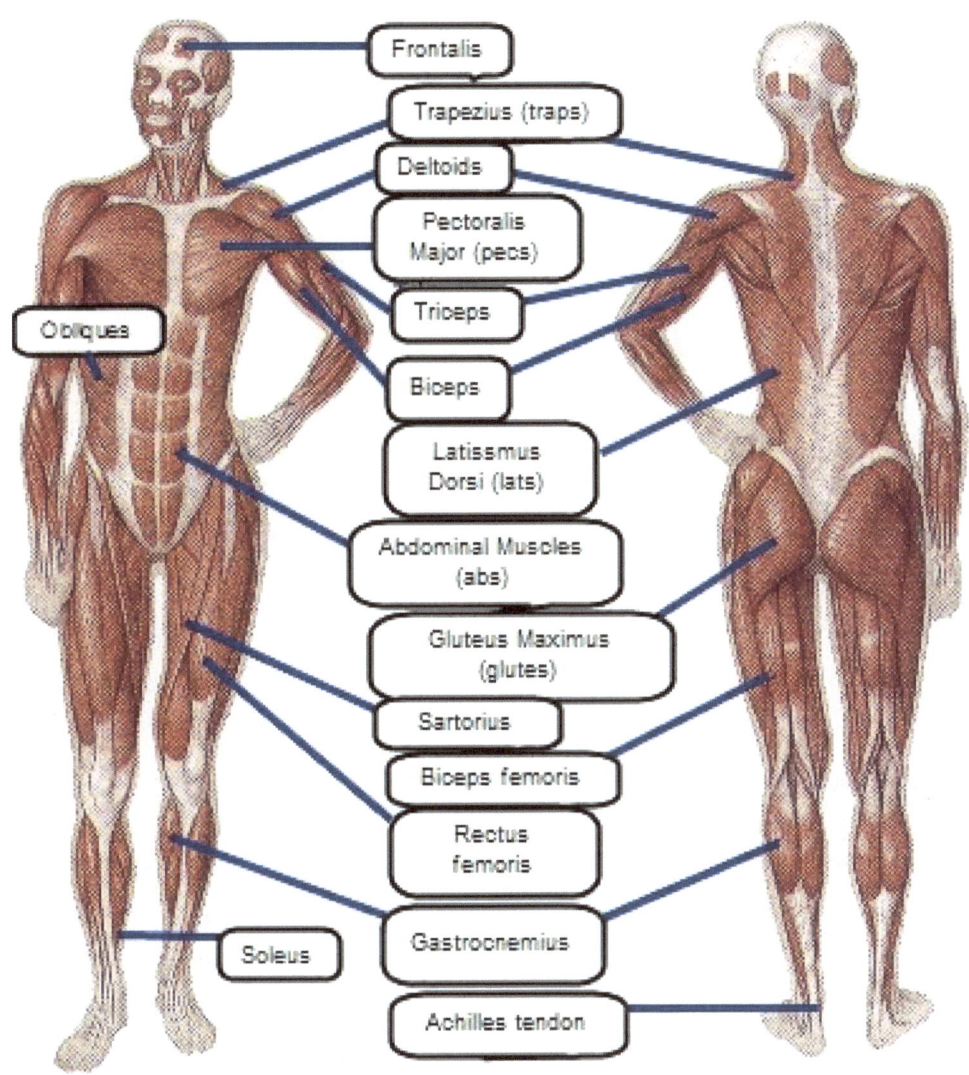

Frontalis

Trapezius (traps)

Deltoids

Pectoralis Major (pecs)

Triceps

Biceps

Latissmus Dorsi (lats)

Obliques

Abdominal Muscles (abs)

Gluteus Maximus (glutes)

Sartorius

Biceps femoris

Rectus femoris

Soleus

Gastrocnemius

Achilles tendon

http://www.fitnesspillars.com/human-body-muscle-diagram.html

Fun Facts about muscles

➢ Hardest muscle in your body is the chin
➢ Strongest muscle in your body is the tongue
➢ You need 17 muscles to smile and 43 to frown
➢ Muscles make up about 40% of your total body weight
➢ The smallest muscles are found in the middle ear
➢ There are more than 600 muscles in your body

Facial muscles

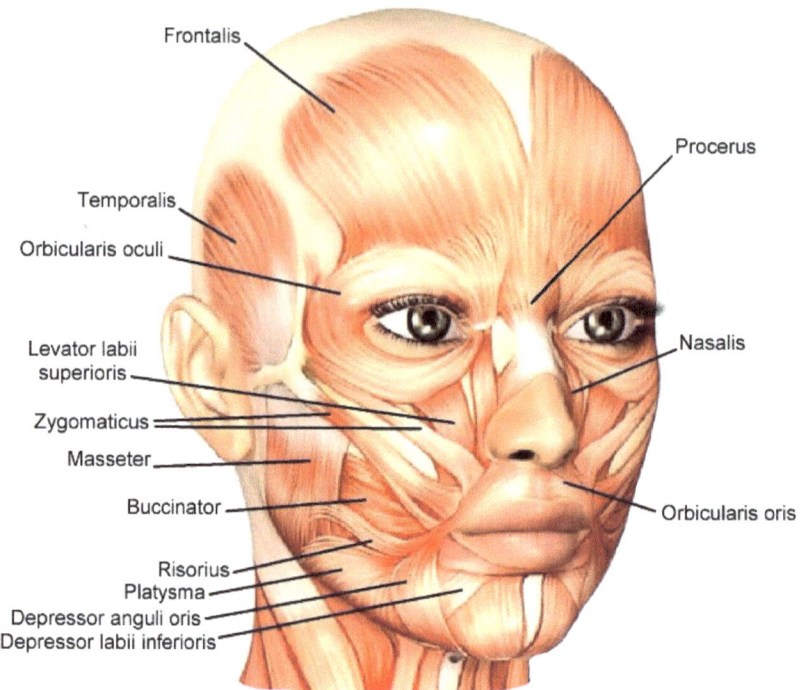

Frontalis

Procerus

Temporalis

Orbicularis oculi

Nasalis

Levator labii
superioris

Zygomaticus

Masseter

Buccinator

Orbicularis oris

Risorius

Platysma

Depressor anguli oris

Depressor labii inferioris

http://devindevon.wikispaces.com/Digestion

Fun Facts about facial muscles

➢ Dimples are caused by short facial muscle
➢ Your face has the biggest range of muscle structure in your body
➢ 43 muscles are directly linked to facial emotions

Skeletal muscle

Fun Facts about skeletal muscles

➢ Produces movement
➢ Maintains posture
➢ Stabilises joints
➢ Generates heat to maintain normal body temperature
➢ Covers your skeleton
➢ Attached to your skeleton by strong, springy tendons
➢ You consciously control what they do
➢ Causes any body movement

Smooth muscle

Fun Facts about smooth muscles

➢ Found in the walls of hollow organs like your intestines and stomach
➢ Work without you being aware of them
➢ Muscular walls of your intestines contract to push food through your body
➢ Smooth muscles in your eyes shrink the size of your pupil

Cardiac muscle

Fun Facts about cardiac muscles

➢ Only exists in your heart
➢ Only type of muscle that doesn't get tired
➢ Contracts to squeeze blood out of your heart; relaxes to fill your heart with blood

Nervous system
Main Nerves

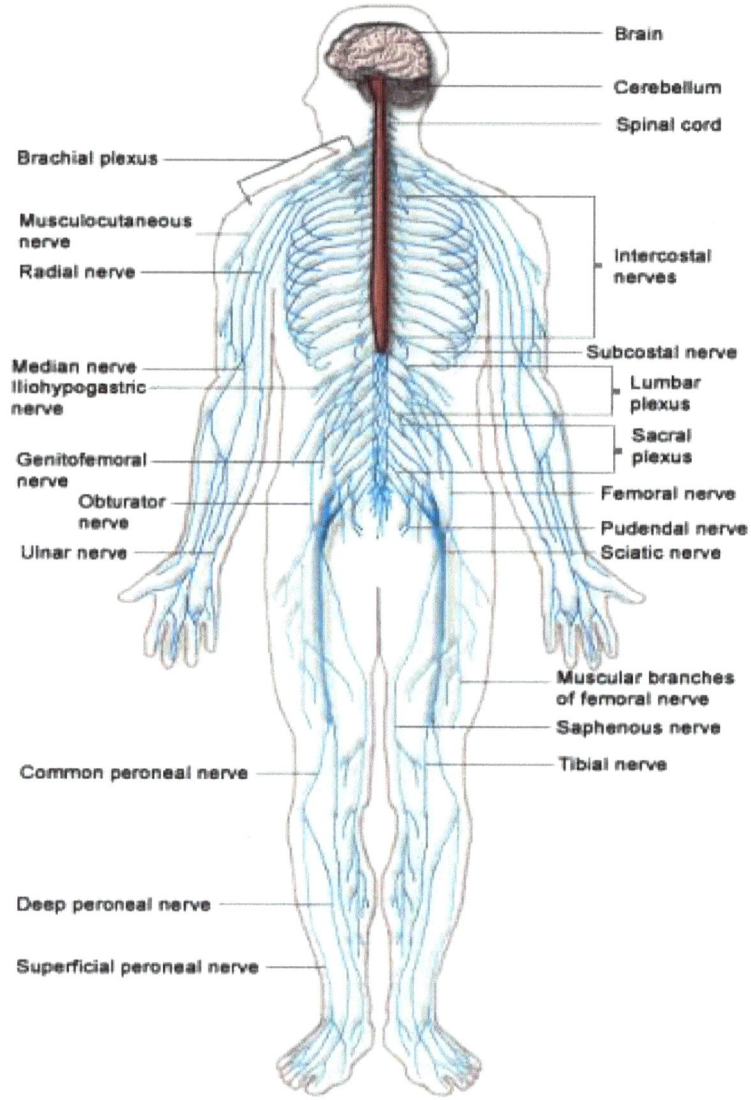

Labels in image:
Brain
Cerebellum
Spinal cord
Brachial plexus
Musculocutaneous nerve
Radial nerve
Intercostal nerves
Median nerve
Iliohypogastric nerve
Subcostal nerve
Lumbar plexus
Sacral plexus
Genitofemoral nerve
Obturator nerve
Femoral nerve
Pudendal nerve
Sciatic nerve
Ulnar nerve
Muscular branches of femoral nerve
Saphenous nerve
Tibial nerve
Common peroneal nerve
Deep peroneal nerve
Superficial peroneal nerve

http://www.ashlandschools.org/morgan_cottle/body/nervous.htm

Fun Facts about nerves

➢ If all your nerves were to be spread out it would be 600 miles long
➢ Can transmit impulses as fast as 100 meters per second
➢ The left side of your brain controls the right side of your body and the right side of your brain controls the left side of your body
➢ Neurons are the largest cells in the human body
➢ Potassium and sodium ions are healthy for your nerves

Spinal cord

brain

NERVES

FUNCTIONS

VERTEBRAE
NUMBERS

Cervical Division

C1
C2
C3
C4
C5
C6
C7
C8

Breathing (C1-4) and
head and neck movement (C2)

Heart rate (C4-6)
and shoulder movement (C5)

Wrist and elbow
movement (C6-7)

Hand and finger
movement (C7-T1)

Thoracic Division

T1
T2
T3
T4
T5
T6
T7
T8
T9
T10
T11
T12

Sympathetic tone (T1-12)
(including temperature regulation)
and trunk stability (T2-12)

Lumbar Division

Sacral Division

L1
L2
L3
L4
L5

Ejaculation (T11-L2)
and hip motion (L2)

Knee extension (L3)

Foot motion (L4-S1)
and knee flexion (L5)

S1
S2
S3
S4
S5

Penile erection (S2-S4)
and bowel and bladder activity (S2-S3)

http://sifoundation.webs.com/spinalcordinjury.htm

Fun Facts about the spinal cord

➢ 18 inches long; 1/4-1/2 of an inch in diameter
➢ Also called medulla spinalis
➢ You have 33 vertabrae in your spine; 9 vertebrae are below the back
➢ You have twelve vertebrae in your thoracic area(the middle portion of the back)
➢ You have five vertebrae in your lumbar spine area(the lower back)
➢ Your neck has seven individual vertebrae

17

Brain

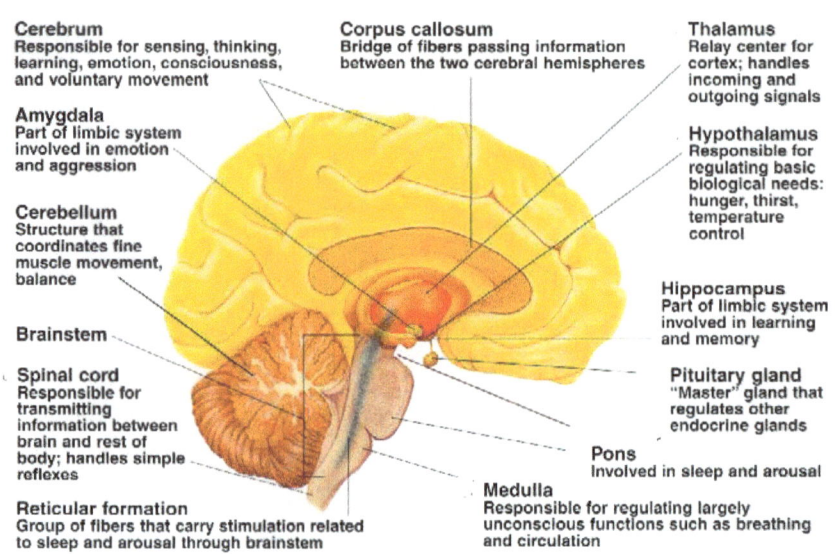

Cerebrum
Responsible for sensing, thinking, learning, emotion, consciousness, and voluntary movement

Amygdala
Part of limbic system involved in emotion and aggression

Cerebellum
Structure that coordinates fine muscle movement, balance

Brainstem

Spinal cord
Responsible for transmitting information between brain and rest of body; handles simple reflexes

Reticular formation
Group of fibers that carry stimulation related to sleep and arousal through brainstem

Corpus callosum
Bridge of fibers passing information between the two cerebral hemispheres

Medulla
Responsible for regulating largely unconscious functions such as breathing and circulation

Pons
Involved in sleep and arousal

Thalamus
Relay center for cortex; handles incoming and outgoing signals

Hypothalamus
Responsible for regulating basic biological needs: hunger, thirst, temperature control

Hippocampus
Part of limbic system involved in learning and memory

Pituitary gland
"Master" gland that regulates other endocrine glands

http://winesurprises.com/brain/the-brain-functions-and-parts.html

Fun Facts about the brain

➢ Your brain weighs about 3 lbs
➢ The cerebrum is the largest part of your brain and weighs 85% of your total brain weight
➢ Gray matter is a tissue in your brain that mainly consists of neurons, which gatherand transmit signals; takes up 40% of your brain
➢ White matter is made up of dendrons and axons, which create a network in which the neurons send signals; takes up 60% of your brain
➢ Water makes up75% of your brain
➢ Your brain consists of about 100 billion neurons
➢ You have 100, 000 miles of blood vessels in your brain
➢ Your brain is the fattest organ in your body

Circulatory System
Main Arteries and Veins

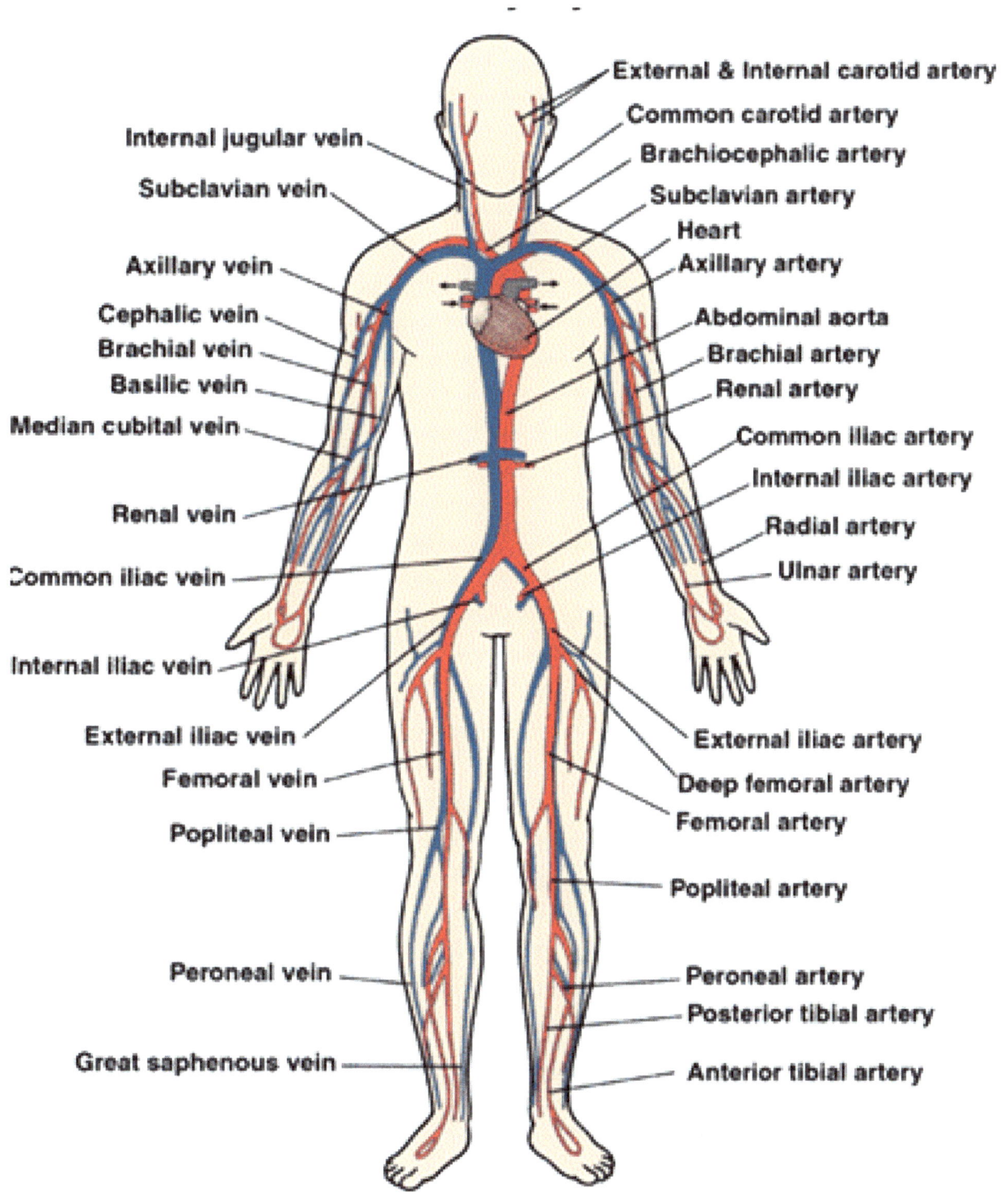

External & Internal carotid artery

Common carotid artery

Brachiocephalic artery

Subclavian artery

Heart

Axillary artery

Abdominal aorta

Brachial artery

Renal artery

Common iliac artery

Internal iliac artery

Radial artery

Ulnar artery

External iliac artery

Deep femoral artery

Femoral artery

Popliteal artery

Peroneal artery

Posterior tibial artery

Anterior tibial artery

Internal jugular vein

Subclavian vein

Axillary vein

Cephalic vein

Brachial vein

Basilic vein

Median cubital vein

Renal vein

Common iliac vein

Internal iliac vein

External iliac vein

Femoral vein

Popliteal vein

Peroneal vein

Great saphenous vein

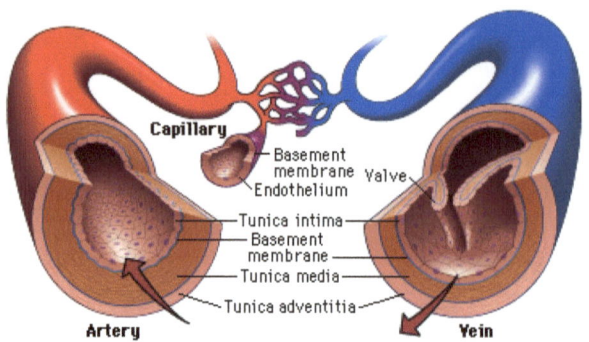

http://www.phschool.com/science/biology_place/biocoach/cardio2/structure.html

Fun Facts about arteries

- ➤ Have thick walls
- ➤ Extra smooth muscle gives them strength and elasticity to deal with surges of blood
- ➤ Most small arterioles don't have thick walls
- ➤ Carries blood away from the heart
- ➤ The pulmonary artery is the only artery that carries deoxygenated blood
- ➤ Tough on the outside; smooth in the inside
- ➤ Deliver oxygen energy and nutrients
- ➤ Carry bright red blood

Fun Facts about veins

- ➤ Prevent blood from backing up
- ➤ Allow some blood to collect without bursting
- ➤ Extra blood is stored in veins
- ➤ Have valves to prevent backflow
- ➤ Wider inner diameters
- ➤ Collects waste
- ➤ Bring blood to the heart
- ➤ Brings reddish blue blood which is low in oxygen

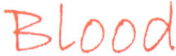

Fun Facts about blood

- ➤ What's in your blood
  55% of plasma
  41% of red blood cells
  4% white blood cells and platelets
- ➤ Take oxygen from lungs and give it to your organs and tissues
- ➤ Different groups of blood: A; B; AB; O
- ➤ 70% of your blood is in veins
- ➤ 20% of your blood is in arteries
- ➤ 10% of your blood is in capillaries
- ➤ Average adult has between 4.7 and 5.0 litres of blood in their body
- ➤ Is a tissue

Heart

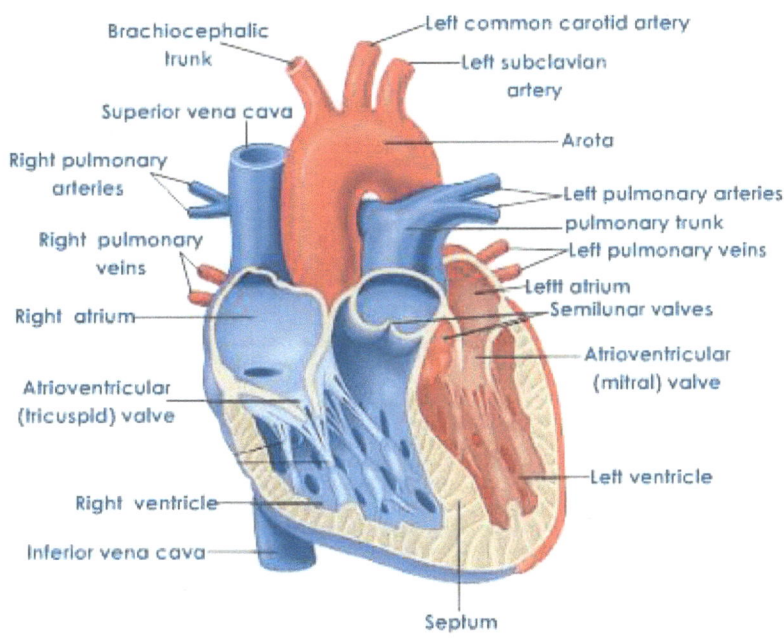

Brachiocephalic trunk
Left common carotid artery
Left subclavian artery
Superior vena cava
Aorta
Right pulmonary arteries
Left pulmonary arteries
pulmonary trunk
Right pulmonary veins
Left pulmonary veins
Left atrium
Semilunar valves
Right atrium
Atrioventricular (mitral) valve
Atrioventricular (tricuspid) valve
Left ventricle
Right ventricle
Inferior vena cava
Septum

http://en.wikipedia.org/wiki/Heart

Heart circulation process

1. Right pump sends blood to the lungs where blood absorbs oxygen
2. Blood goes to the left pump where it is pumped to the rest of thebody

Fun Facts about heart

➢ Has 2 pumps
➢ Sends 1/3 cup of blood for each pump
➢ Beats 70 times a minute
➢ Weighs 11 oz on average
➢ Pumps 2,000 gallons of blood through blood vessels each day
➢ A female's heart beats faster than a male's
➢ Your heart starts beating after you are 4 weeks old and doesn't stop until you die

Fun Facts about Blood Vessels

➢ There are 62,000 miles in your whole body
➢ One drop would take a minute to travel your whole body

Respiratory System
Main Organs

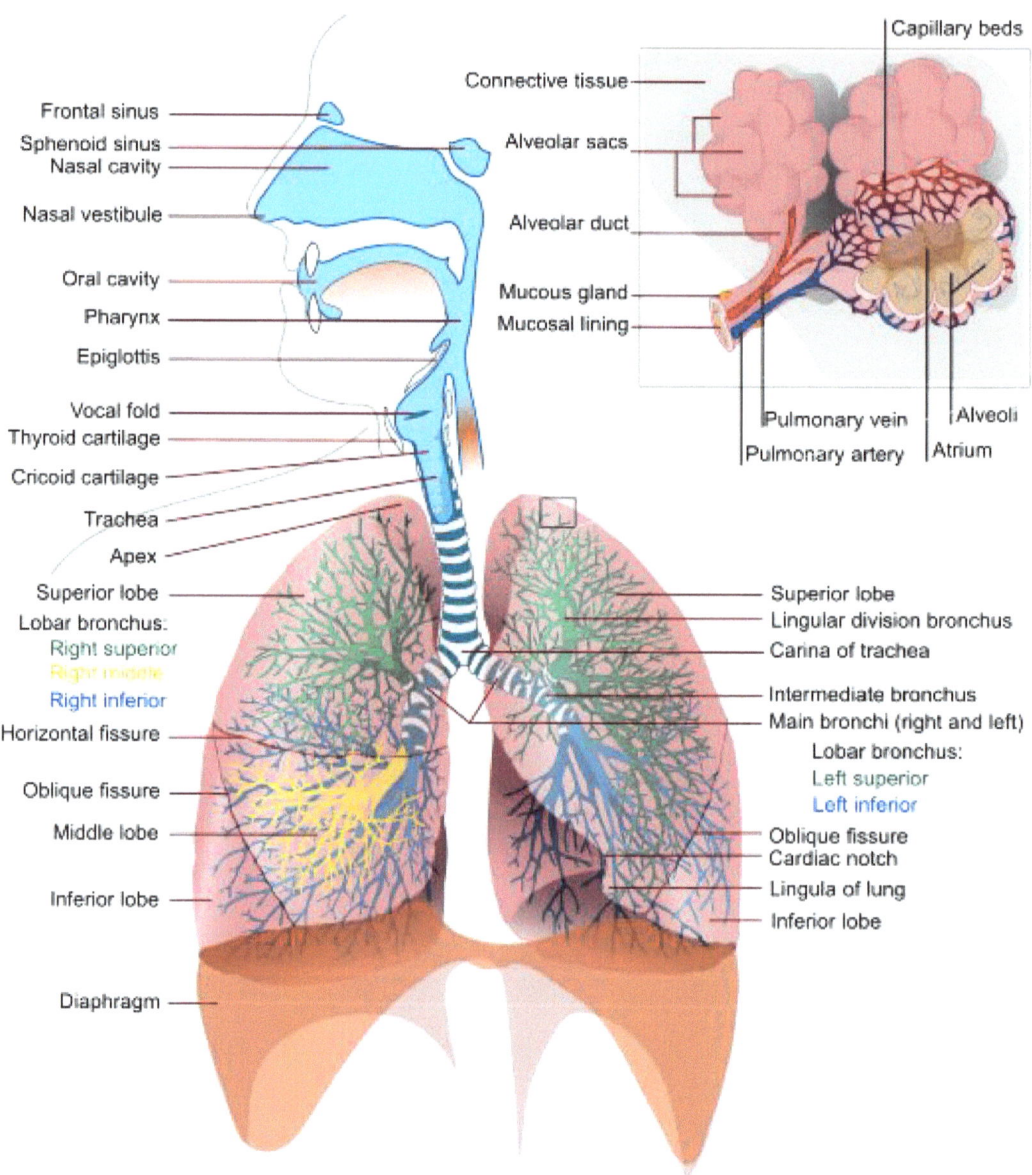

http://www.healthguideinfo.com/respiratory-conditions/p57144/

Fun Facts about respiratory

➢ About 2 cups of air flows in/out for each breath
➢ Hiccups are caused by sudden movements in diaphragm

Breathing

Breathing Process

1. Air is sucked in from the nose into lungs
2. Lungs expand
3. Ribs move up and out
4. Diaphram pulls down and out
5. Diaphram curves up
6. Intercostals, muscles and space in between the ribs, relax
7. Ribs move down and in
8. Lungs contract
9. Air is pushed out

fun facts about breathing process

➢ Air has 21% oxygen, but your body only needs 5% of it
➢ Breathing through your mouth shrinks your jaw
➢ You change sides in our sleep about every 30 minutes because you are balancing beathing through each of the nostrils

Lungs

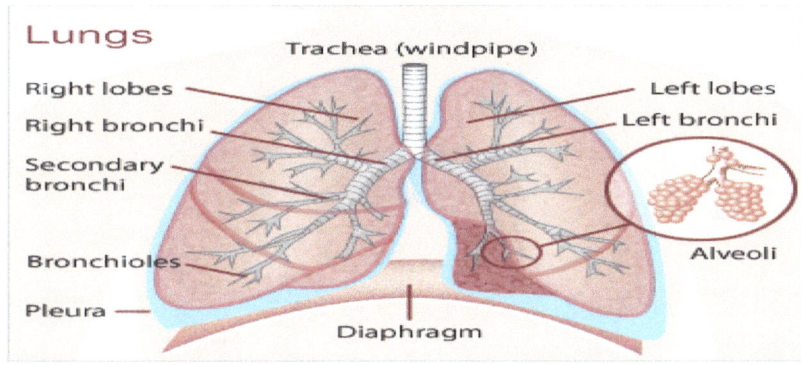

http://tcmdiscovery.com/BasicTheoryofTCM/info/20130528_16865.html

fun facts about lungs

➢ Your lung on your left side is smaller than your right
➢ Consists of over 300,000 million capillaries, or tiny blood vessels; if they were to be spread out they would be 1,500 miles long
➢ If your lungs were open flat they would cover the size of a tennis court
➢ Alveoli is a passageway that allows air to go to the blood
➢ You have approximately 300 to 400 million alveoli in each lung that are mainly found in "pockets" of your lungs
➢ Your lungs act like air filters in a cars

Voice Box or trachea

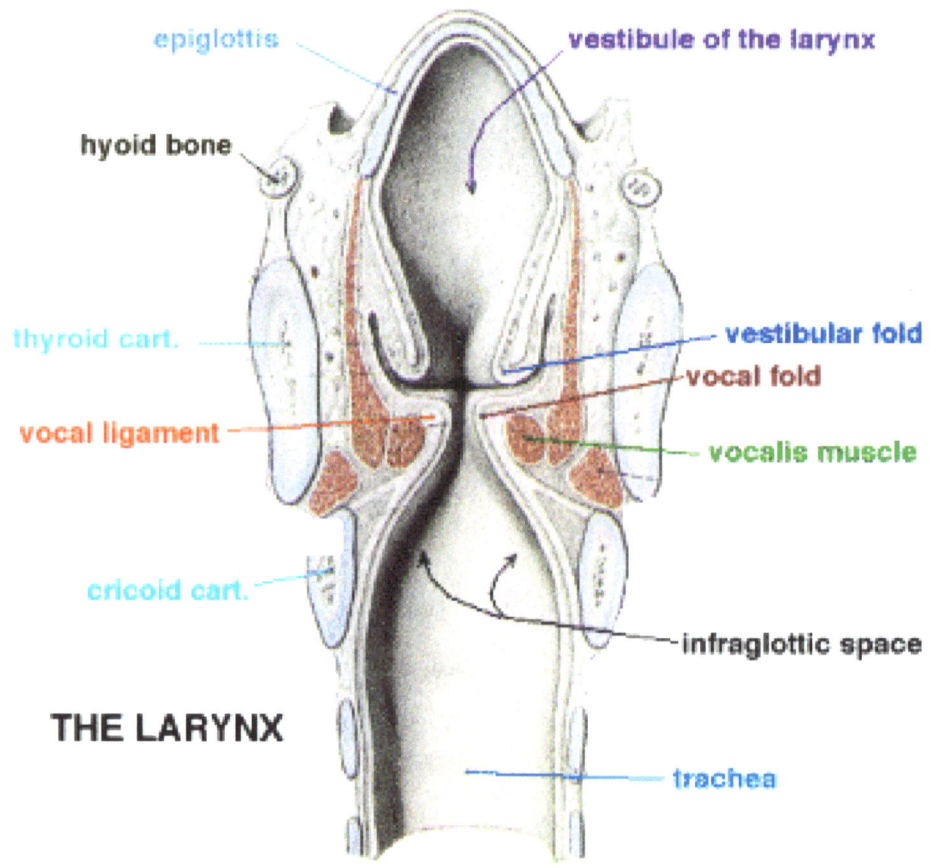

THE LARYNX

Labels: epiglottis, vestibule of the larynx, hyoid bone, thyroid cart., vestibular fold, vocal fold, vocal ligament, vocalis muscle, cricoid cart., infraglottic space, trachea

http://freesingingvoice.blogspot.com/

fun facts about voice box

- ➤ Can be called larynx
- ➤ Made of 9 plates of cartilage
- ➤ Allow you to make sounds
- ➤ Vocal cords are basically are folds that are made up of different layers of muscles, ligaments, and membrane
- ➤ Whispering can make your vocal cords work harder
- ➤ Many of your muscles used for swallowing are also used for talking
- ➤ Sinuses are airfilled spaces off the nasal cavity that help make different sounds of speech
- ➤ Women's voices are higher because their vocal cords are shorter and vibrate more quickly
- ➤ Men's vocal cord are 2/3-1 inch long
- ➤ Women's vocal cord is 1/2-2/3 inch long

Nose (breathing)

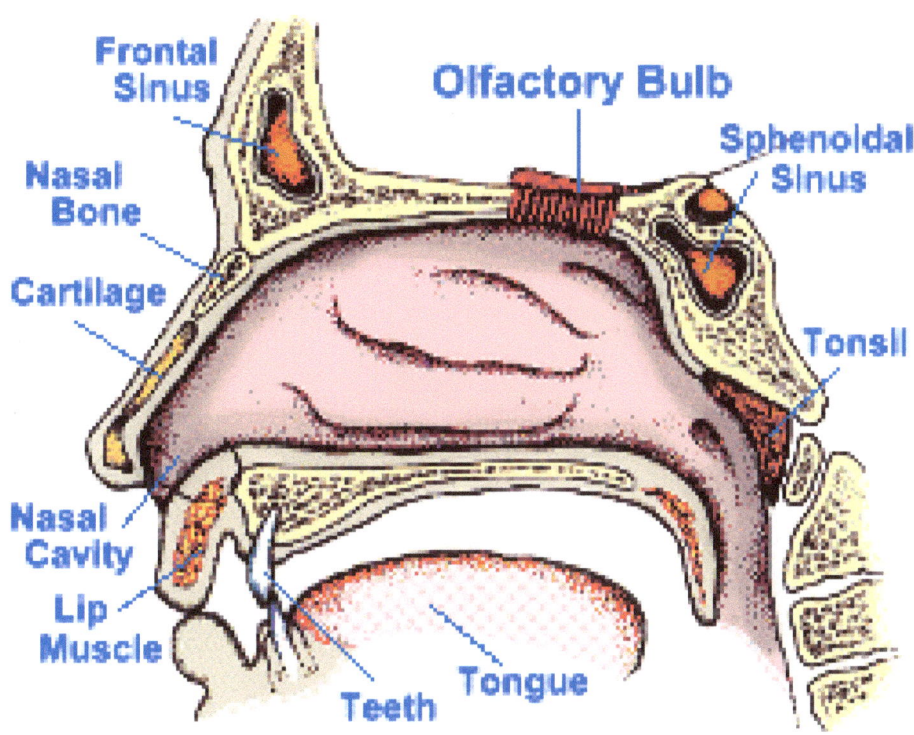

http://petro256.wordpress.com/

fun facts about nose

➢ Has hair that catches dust and other small particles
➢ 2 nostrils work as air filters
➢ Has special cells that help you smell
➢ 2 nostrils are divided by the nasal septum
➢ Nasal septum is made of cartilage
➢ Air passes through the nose and is changed to the right temperature
➢ The floor of your nasal cavity is also the roof of your mouth

Digestive System

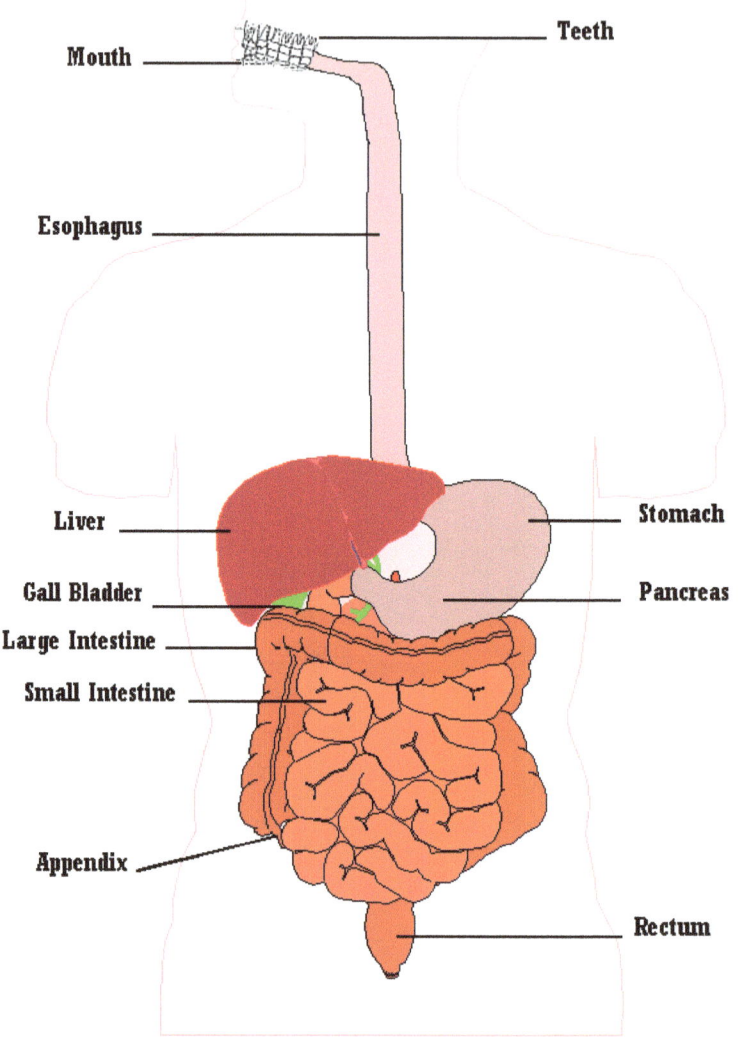

Mouth

Teeth

Esophagus

Liver

Stomach

Gall Bladder

Pancreas

Large Intestine

Small Intestine

Appendix

Rectum

http://digestion.ism-online.org/category/pancreas-and-kidneys/

Digestion Process

- ➤ Food is chewed by teeth; saliva breaks down the carbohydrates in the food; 1 minute
- ➤ Food is swallowed down the throat (5-10 sec) and is pushed down the esophagus into the stomach
- ➤ Food is put into a ball, called chyme in the somach; 1-3 hours
- ➤ Chyme goes through the small and large intestine; 12-36 hours
- ➤ Waste is passes down the anus

Fun facts about the Digestion Process

- ➤ Converts food into nutrients your body needs
- ➤ Gets rid of the body of waste
- ➤ Food doesn't need gravity to get to your stomach

Teeth

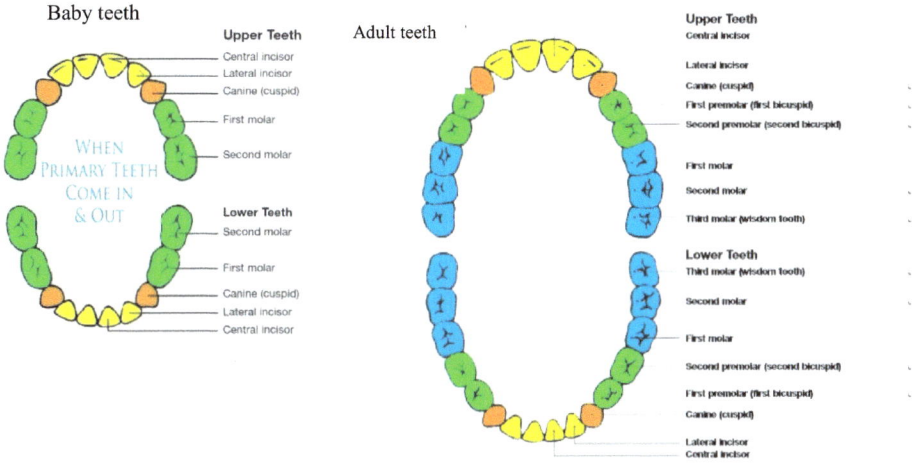

Teeth Order http://comfortdds.com/dentist-lafayette-in/dentistry-by-stage/tooth-schedule/

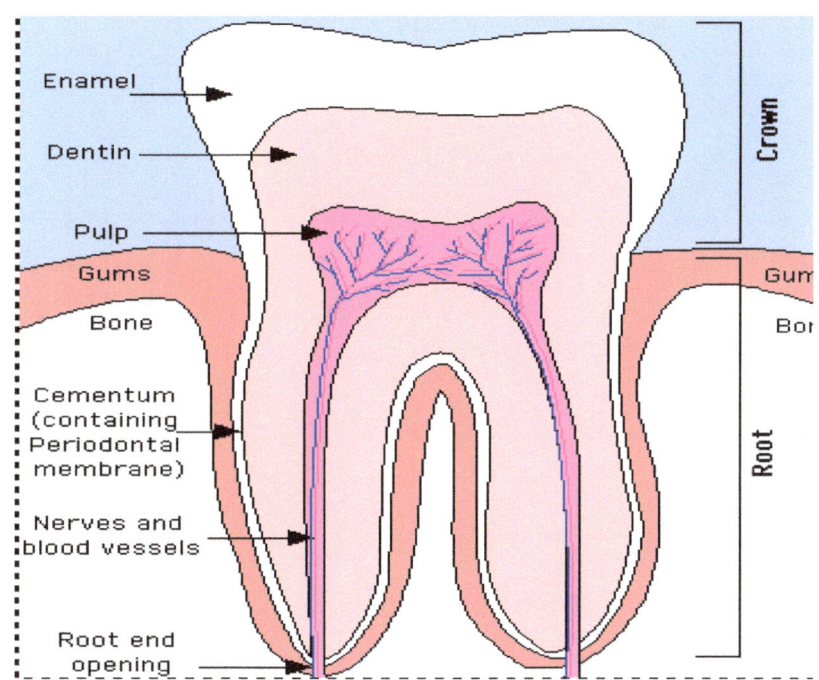

Tooth Structure http://www.enchantedlearning.com/subjects/anatomy/teeth/toothlabeled.GIF

Fun facts about teeth

➢ 2 parts of a tooth: crown above gum; roots below gum
➢ Crown is made of enamel
➢ Roots supply tooth with nutrients

Stomach

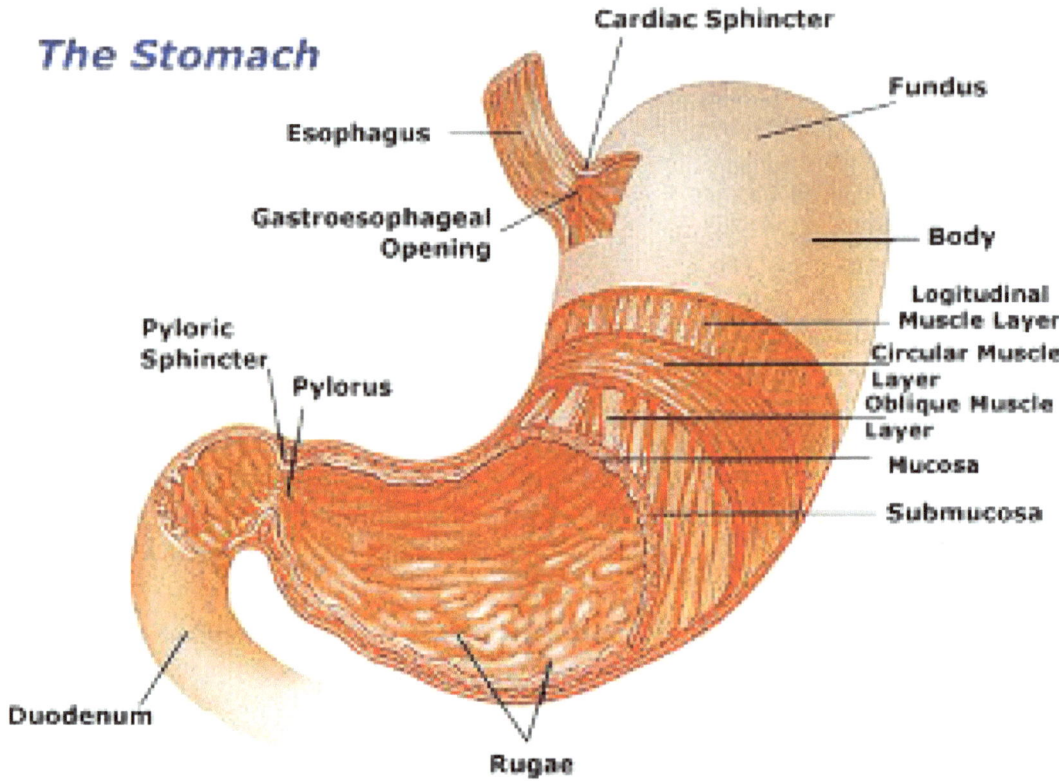

The Stomach

Fun facts about stomach

- ➢ Sits below left lung
- ➢ Made of smooth muscle
- ➢ Smooth muscle squeezes the food in your stomach
- ➢ In the stomach there is hydrochloric acid which kills all bacteria
- ➢ Elastic
- ➢ Located between the esophagus and intestines
- ➢ 12 inches long and 6 inches wide at its most
- ➢ Capcity of an adult is 1qt.
- ➢ Cardiac sphinter is the connection between the esophagus and stomach

Small and Large Intestine

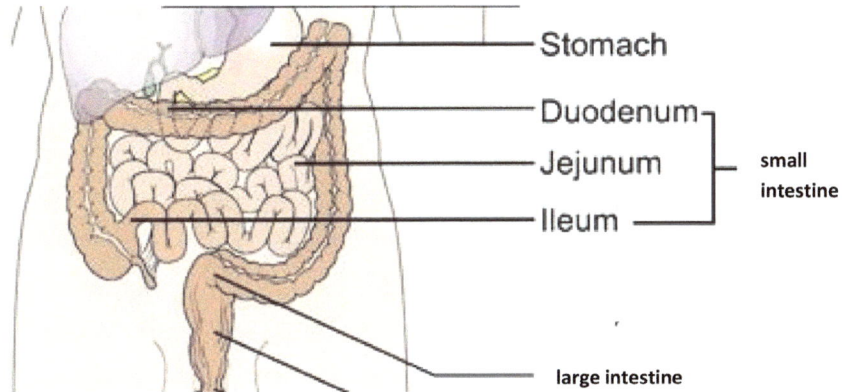

Fun facts about small intestine

➢ 3 parts: duodenum; jejunum; ileum
➢ 20 ft long; longest part of the digestive tract
➢ Coiled
➢ Duodenum: takes semi-digested food from the stomach and helps digest a little bit
➢ Jejunum: carries food to the ilieum
➢ Ileum: where most of nutrients are absorbed before the chyme goes to the large intestine
➢ Receives 1-3 gallons of mashed up food that is in liquid form
➢ Surface area is 25,000 sq feet
➢ Surface is folded
➢ Villi helps absorbs nutrients and is on the surface

Fun facts about large intestine

➢ Around small intestine
➢ 5 ft long
➢ 2-2 1/2 inches wide
➢ Job is to absorb water and salts from the material that has not been digested as food, and to get rid of any waste products left over
➢ Parts are cecum and colon
➢ Cecum takes absorbed liquids from the ileum to the colon
➢ Colon has 4 main parts
➢ Whole colon reabsorbs water, and absorbs salts when needed

Senses

Eyes

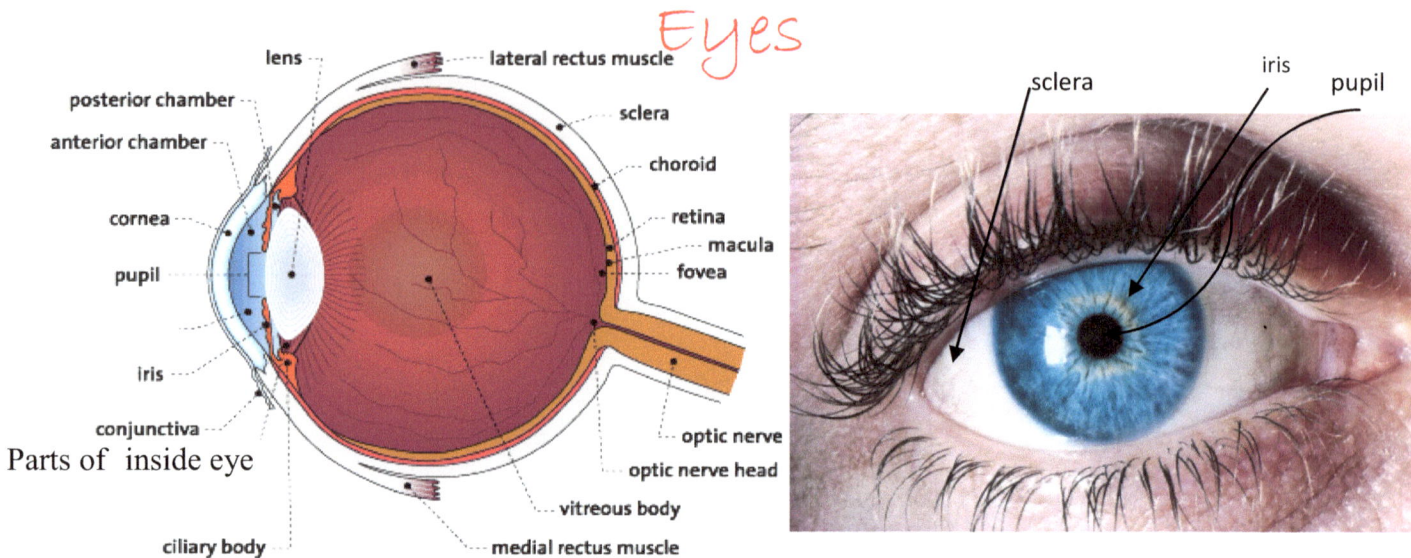

Parts of inside eye

http://www.med.upenn.edu/cpob/studies/studies_site.shtml

Parts of outside eye

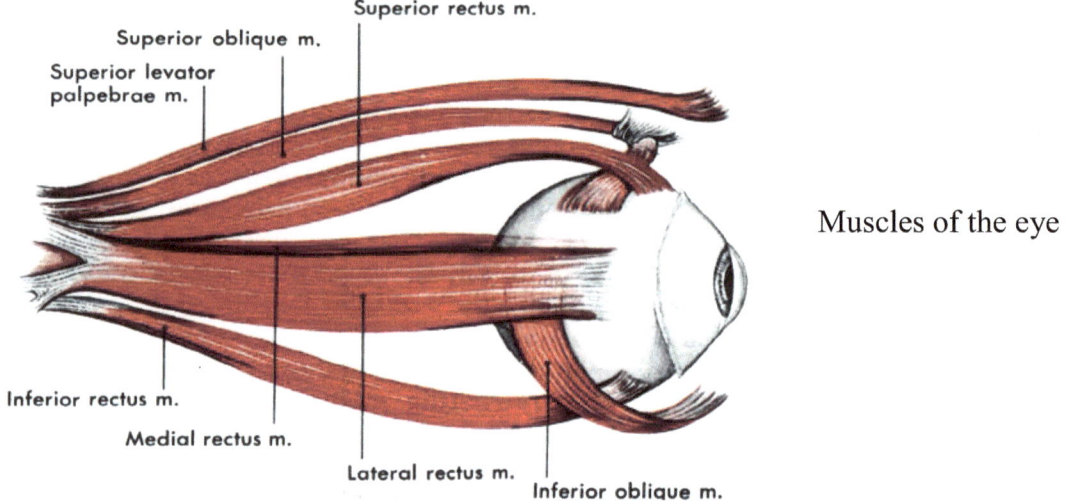

Muscles of the eye

https://students.washington.edu/mjbrooks/gaze-print-biometric-security/eye-muscles-4/

Fun facts about eyes

- ➤ the pupil grows when in dim light and srinks when in bright light
- ➤ your eye is the only part in your body that doesn't grow
- ➤ things you see are sent to your brain by the optic nerve
- ➤ your retina is a light detecting muscle in the inner surface
- ➤ cornea, a lining on the iris and pupil with the lens, refracts light to the retina
- ➤ cone cells in your retina detect color
- ➤ rod cells in your retina detect low light contrasts

Ears

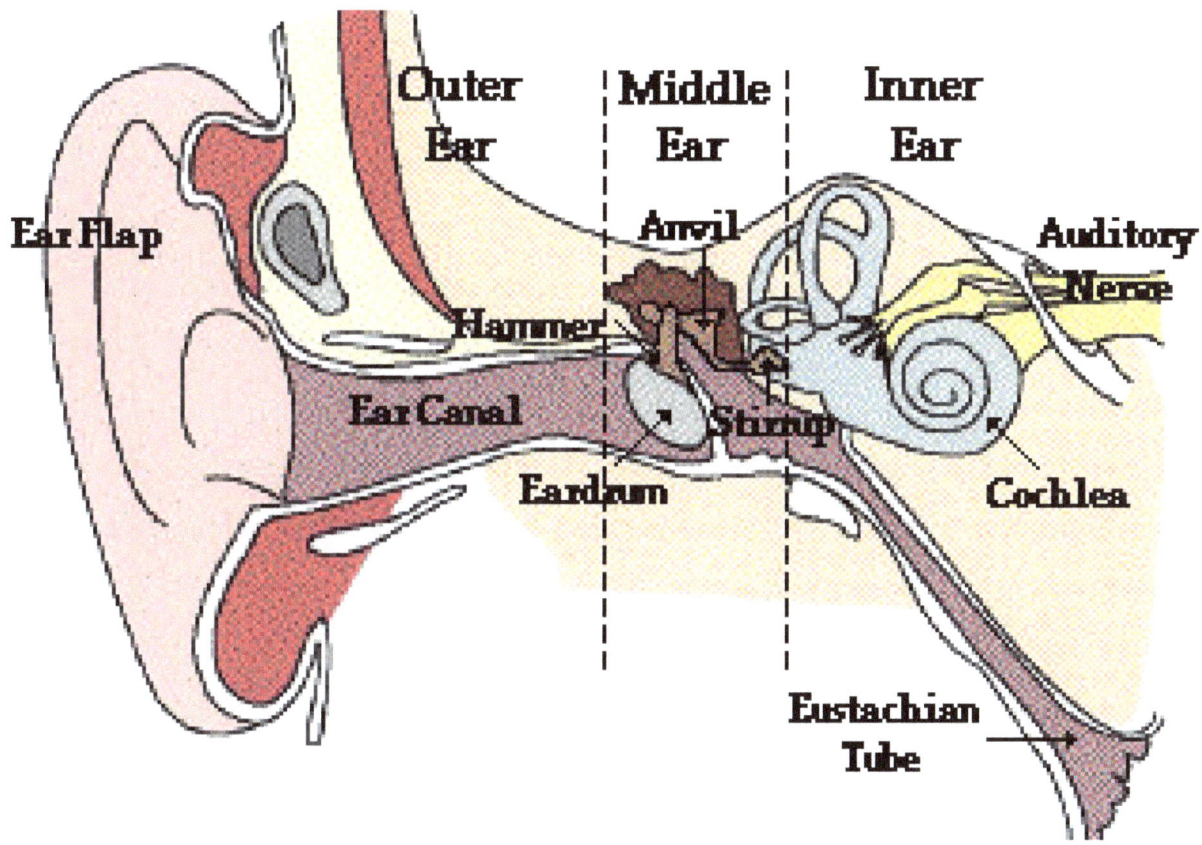

Fun facts about ears

➢ 3 main parts: outer, middle, and inner
➢ Outer part: ear flap,which is outside, and ear canal, which is inside
➢ Middle part: eardrum and 3 small bone(smallest in your whole body)
➢ Inner part: auditory nerve, cochlea, eustachian tube
➢ Convert sound waves into nerve impulses that are sent to the brain through the auditory nerve
➢ Middle part amplifies sound pressure
➢ The temporal bone(found in your ear) is the hardest bone in your body
➢ Abnormalties in your ear can cause deafness
➢ A sound pitch is measured in hertz; the range your ear can hear is 25,000-20,000
➢ Your eardrum has the smallest bone in you body

Nose(smelling)

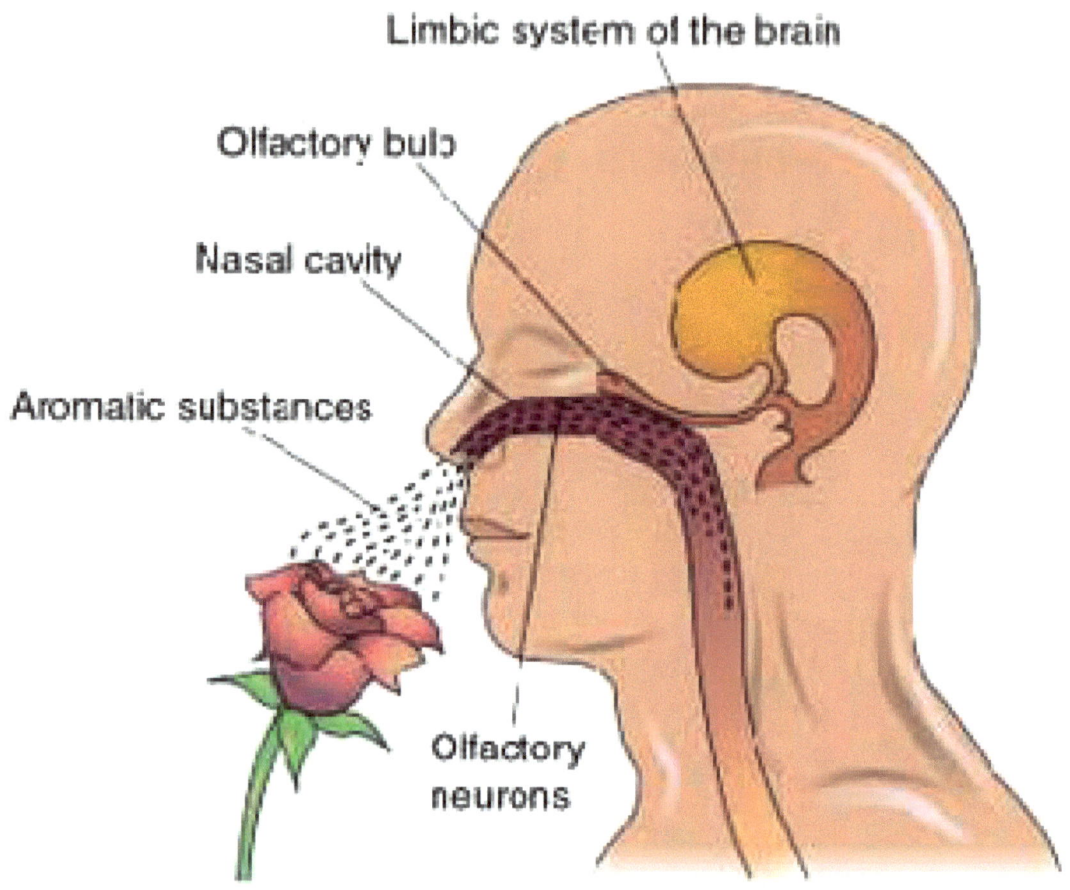

Fun facts about nose

- The scents you are smelling have small particles. These particles land on sensors on the roof of your nasal chamber. The patches of sensors send information about the aroma to your brain
- Women's sense of smell is better than men's
- You have 350 oflactory receptor genes
- Your nose can tell the difference between 10,000 scents

Tongue

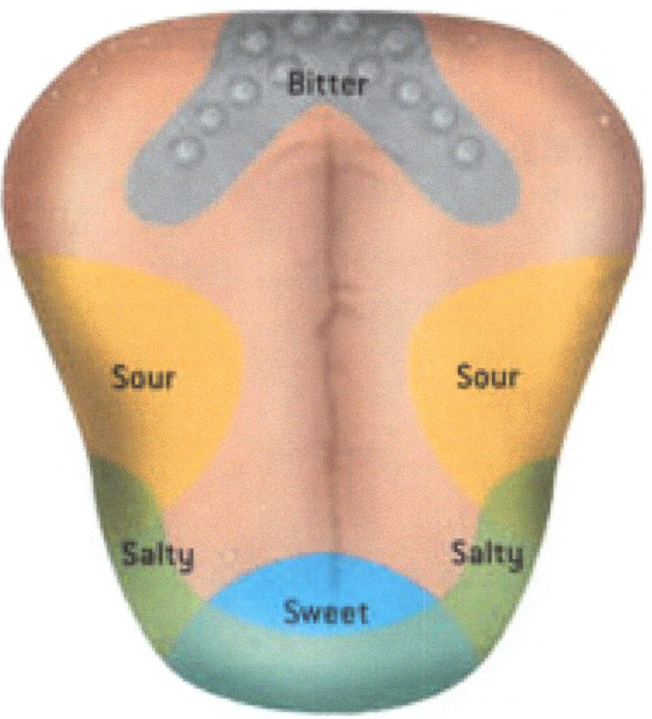

Fun facts about tongue

- ➤ Has papillae(small bumps) used to grip on food
- ➤ Chilies have a strong chemical that makes it taste spicy
- ➤ Over years, some tastebuds die, but are never replaced
- ➤ The center of your tongue has no taste buds
- ➤ Women have shorter tongues than men
- ➤ Your tongue imprint is unique just like your fingerprint
- ➤ An average person has 10,000 taste buds and 2,000 are underneath the tongue
- ➤ Your tongue is your toughest muscle in your body

Acknowledgements

- Arunasri and Dr. Sesha ---- My Parents
- Prof. Srikanth Singamaneni
- Drs. Venkat and Sunitha Dharmavarapu
- Mrs. Kathy Gavin ------ Science teacher
- Google
- Google Images
- http://www.softschools.com/facts/human_body/the_stomach_facts/341/
- http://breath.ygoy.com/2010/06/09/fun-facts-about-respiratory-system/
- http://www.sciencekids.co.nz/